GUIDE ON JOINT PAIN FOR SENIORS

The Effective Natural Remedies to Heal Up and Reduce Arthritis

TABLE OF CONTENT

PREFACE

In the course of our older years, joint discomfort becomes an especially poignant universal burden. Wear and tear on our once-robust joints is an unavoidable consequence of aging, which can be both a boon and a challenge. The discomfort, stiffness, and inflammation that accompany this change cast a pall over daily routines that were formerly simple pleasures, including walking, getting dressed, and even taking a shower.

Common treatments for joint pain include taking painkillers, visiting a doctor, and engaging in physical therapy. Many people, however, are looking for alternatives because they know that this path is fraught with dangers and adverse effects.

Elderly people looking for peace in the embrace of natural medicines will find a beacon of understanding and comfort in the following chapters. This book is a testimonial to the healing power of nature and its inherent wonders. The origins of the joint pain that inevitably comes with old age are explored, and a variety of natural therapies that have been shown to alleviate pain and improve joint function are presented.

The treatments advocated here have been used successfully for generations, and their effectiveness has stood the test of time. They are living proof of their effectiveness and safety, and they can work in tandem with conventional medicine if that's what the patient prefers.

This book is a reliable companion for seniors who are navigating the complex maze of joint discomfort. It provides a wide variety of natural treatments, a treasure trove of knowledge carefully crafted to ease suffering and foster a life full of vitality.

INTRODUCTION

My own parents' dogged struggle with debilitating joint pain served as a catalyst for writing this book. I have seen my parents' health deteriorate over the years as they have struggled with joint discomfort. They were formerly very dynamic and self-reliant, but as their suffering increased, they found themselves increasingly constrained. It broke my heart to watch them stutter and fall when they attempted the simplest of tasks, like getting dressed or out of bed.

They showed unwavering will to not just survive but thrive through endless days that dawned with pain, stiffness, and inflammation. Everyday activities like walking, which most of us do without thinking, became herculean struggles against the constraints imposed by their own joints. Their search for relief took us along traditional medical avenues, illuminating the intricacies and difficulties that many elderly people face along the way. Nothing I did brought them any relief, and I tried everything. The pain was too severe for OTC meds, and the risks associated with prescription drugs were unacceptable. Physical treatment was time-consuming and costly, but it did help a little. The desire for a solution that fits in with the natural harmony of life became deeper alongside the frustration of restricted possibilities and unexpected adverse effects.

Seeing the challenges my parents faced inspired me to make it my life's work to collect the advice and insights that will help other seniors find the peace of mind, freedom of movement, and renewed vigor that my parents had in their latter years. This book is an homage to my parents, who inspired me to keep looking for a better life via their strength, perseverance, and undying love.

This book was written to disseminate the homeopathic treatments that alleviated my mother's arthritis. I'm hoping it will be useful for other elderly people dealing with the same issue. While crippling pain in the joints is common, it need not be permanent. There are pain-relieving and joint-enhancing natural therapies available. I'm writing this book in the hopes that it would give elderly people hope that they can find comfort and have fuller, pain-free lives."

CHAPTER ONE

Joint Pain Overview

For many elderly people, joint discomfort is a continuous companion that has been with them throughout history. Herbal treatments, yoga positions, and mindful practices were just some of the holistic approaches that people from all walks of life employed in the past to alleviate joint pain. These techniques are still used today to alleviate joint pain, and they originated in the notion that one's body, mind, and soul are all interconnected.

Joint pain conditions including osteoarthritis and rheumatoid arthritis have been better understood since the development of modern medicine. This resulted in the creation of cutting-edge medical interventions like antibiotics, surgical procedures, and rehabilitative exercises. Joint discomfort is a common problem for the elderly, but many are now turning to complementary holistic approaches in addition to conventional medical care. The theory behind this strategy is that treating symptoms rather than the underlying causes of joint pain is more effective in the long run.

Seniors' joint discomfort has a long and fascinating history, one marked by tenacity, creativity, and a never-ending search for alleviation.

People have long discovered ways to deal with joint discomfort and carry on with meaningful lives, from traditional natural treatments to cutting-edge medical advances. Now more than ever, elderly people with joint discomfort have a wide variety of options from which to pick. And you're on the verge of seeing all the mysteries you've been missing!

How Arthritis Hurts

Arthritis and associated disorders come in more than a hundred distinct varieties. Osteoarthritis (OA), Rheumatoid Arthritis (RA), Psoriatic Arthritis (PsA), Fibromyalgia, and Gout are the most typical forms. Debilitating, life-altering pain can be caused by arthritis and related disorders in a variety of ways.

Osteoarthritis

Degenerative joint disease osteoarthritis (OA) causes discomfort and difficulty moving affected joints as lubricating cartilage and fluid deteriorate over time. At some point, the bones of the joint may begin to rub directly against one another. Knees, hips, hands, and spines are the most common sites of OA manifestation, and inflammation plays a role in the disease's progression. Different people experience pain at different levels. It may be treatable with medication and frequent physical activity for mild to moderate cases.

Some people are severely afflicted by it, to the point where even the slightest motion of the affected joint is excruciating.

Pain and inflammation can be mitigated with the help of nonsteroidal anti-inflammatory medications (NSAIDs). In some cases, acetaminophen (Tylenol) alone can relieve pain just as well as nonsteroidal anti-inflammatory drugs (NSAIDs), but with fewer GI side effects. Acetaminophen is found in many over-the-counter drugs; however, ingesting too much of it can be harmful to the liver. Consult your doctor about other treatments if your OA pain is severe and ongoing. In extreme circumstances, joint replacement surgery may be the only viable option.

People with OA have found great benefit from non-pharmaceutical pain management. Hot and cold packs, topical rubs, and physical therapy are all examples of such treatments.

Rheumatoid Arthritis and Juvenile Idiopathic Arthritis

Rheumatoid arthritis (RA) occurs when the immune system mistakenly assaults healthy tissue in the body, including the joints and other organs. Inflammation is generally triggered by the immune system to defend the body from harmful pathogens.

The synovium, the lining of the joints, is attacked by inflammation that becomes hyperactive in persons with autoimmune illnesses like RA. Joint and other organ damage from ongoing inflammation can be permanent and progressively painful.

Usually, RA strikes symmetrical joints, like both knees or both hands. The liver, heart, and eyes are only some of the internal organs that can be harmed. The process in juvenile idiopathic arthritis (JIA) works similarly to that in RA, but it's important to note that JIA is not a child-sized version of RA. Similar to RA, it can spread beyond the joints and harm the internal organs and eyes. Disease flares, in which patients with RA or JIA experience a temporary worsening of symptoms like pain, are common among those who suffer from these conditions. Disease-modifying antirheumatic medications (DMARDs) and biologics, which are used to treat the diseases itself, are often successful at reducing pain as well.

Psoriatic Arthritis

Psoriatic arthritis (PsA), like rheumatoid arthritis (RA) and juvenile idiopathic arthritis (JIA), is an autoimmune inflammatory illness that mostly affects the skin and joints. Psoriasis sufferers are more likely to have this condition, as the rapid turnover of skin cells is a hallmark of this autoimmune illness.

These areas may itch or hurt, and if left untreated they may dry out and crack, which is quite uncomfortable.

The joints are not immune to PsA. It may also have an effect on the entheses, or the points at which ligaments and tendons join to bones. Common sites of enthesitis inflammation include the lower back and the bottom of the foot. Pain relief may be achieved by using DMARDs or biologics for PsA treatment. Psoriasis patients may benefit from further dermatologist care.

Fibromyalgia

The malfunction of the brain and spinal cord in fibromyalgia is thought to be the root of the condition, making it a disorder of chronic pain. Pain throughout the body is a hallmark of fibromyalgia, and it can be intermittent or chronic. Pain signals may be heightened in fibromyalgia due to amplification of central nervous system impulses. Because of a condition called allodynia, even the slightest touch or movement can be excruciatingly painful for someone with fibromyalgia, and hyperalgesia can make even the mildest pain intolerable.

Pain perception may also be exacerbated by other symptoms such as weariness, sleeplessness, inattention, and emotional distress.

Antidepressants and anticonvulsants (like Lyrica) are two examples of neurochemical-targeting pharmaceuticals used in treatment. Exercise and acupuncture are two examples of non-drug treatments that have shown promise.

Gout

While inflammatory conditions like RA and PsA lead to systemic swelling, gout does not have this effect. The cause of gout is excess uric acid in the body. Excess uric acid can develop crystals in joints if the body produces too much of it or if it is not removed quickly enough (a condition known as hyperuricemia). The resulting inflammation of the joints is very painful. If left untreated, these crystals can grow into painful lumps (tophi) in the afflicted joint or the tissues around it. The big toe joint is where gout most frequently manifests, but it can affect any joint. A gout flare can cause you to feel fine before night, but then wreak havoc on your day.

Anti-inflammatory drugs, corticosteroids, and colchicine, an anti-gout medication, are used to treat the initial flare. After an acute attack of gout has subsided, uric acid-lowering medications are used to keep the condition under control.

Preventing future outbreaks of gout can also be accomplished by making adjustments to one's lifestyle, such as drinking more water and avoiding alcohol and purine-rich meals.

Lupus

Joints, kidneys, skin, blood, the brain, and other organs are just some of the places where lupus, also known as systemic lupus erythematosus (SLE), can wreak havoc. Symptoms range from weariness to hair loss to sensitivity to light to fever to a rash to renal issues to discomfort in the joints or chest. Lupus is treated with a wide range of drugs because its manifestations vary from person to person. Anti-inflammatory drugs, DMARDs, and corticosteroids are just a few examples. Anti-TNF medications belimumab (Benlysta) and anifrolumab (Saphnelo) are the only ones currently approved to treat lupus.

Back Pain

Ankylosing spondylitis, psoriatic arthritis, spinal stenosis, and fibromyalgia are all forms of arthritis that can cause back discomfort, one of the most common reasons people visit their doctor. However, most cases of back discomfort can be traced back to an incident that involved an injury, such as incorrect lifting or bending, a sports injury, or a car crash. Heat and cold, exercise, and stress management are all examples of nondrug treatments. In addition to

DMARDs, analgesics, and even biologics, nonsteroidal anti-inflammatory drugs (NSAIDs) may be used for pain relief.

CHAPTER TWO

Nutrition and Diet

The role of anti-inflammatory foods in joint health

The ability to move freely and easily depends on joints, which are complex linkages between bones. Joint discomfort and limited mobility can be the result of both age-related wear and tear and the development of chronic inflammation. The link between nutrition and joint health is especially important for the elderly because inflammation has such a profound effect on joint health. This highlights the importance of the idea of employing anti-inflammatory foods to enhance joint health.

While inflammation is an important part of the body's defense system, it can cause more harm than good if it persists for too long. The aging process and other factors increase the risk of chronic inflammation in the elderly. Joint disorders like osteoarthritis and rheumatoid arthritis can be made worse by chronic inflammation, which can cause pain, stiffness, and a decline in quality of life.

In the fight against inflammation and its consequences on the joints of the elderly, several minerals have emerged as potent allies.

Anti-inflammatory omega-3 fatty acids are found in abundance in oily fish like salmon, flaxseeds, and walnuts. These fatty acids contribute to a healthy inflammatory response in the body, which may lessen joint discomfort and improve joint function.

The antioxidants that are so abundant in fresh, vibrant produce become increasingly important as we get older. They help prevent inflammation and tissue damage by neutralizing free radicals. Minerals like selenium and zinc, as well as vitamins C and E, are essential in preventing damage to joint tissues caused by oxidative stress.

As they age, the importance of vitamin D, which is essential for bone health and inflammatory regulation, increases. In order to reduce inflammation and promote joint function in the elderly, it is important to keep vitamin D levels at optimal levels through sun exposure, fortified meals, and supplements.

The key to an anti-inflammatory diet for the elderly is making conscious decisions that benefit joint health. The anti-inflammatory benefits of a diet rich in whole grains, lean proteins, legumes, nuts, seeds, and a wide variety of fruits and vegetables are manifold. with addition to providing essential nutrients, these foods also aid with skeletal mobility and comfort.

While there is a lot of focus on anti-inflammatory foods, it's also vital for seniors to avoid eating things that may cause inflammation.

Inflammation can be made worse by consuming processed foods, too much sugar, or trans fats. In order to control inflammation and promote senior joint health, finding a healthy balance between pro-inflammatory and anti-inflammatory diets is essential.

Seniors are given the tools they need to take charge of their health as they embark on the path toward sustaining joint health with anti-inflammatory nutrition. Seniors may improve their inflammation, joint discomfort, and quality of life by eating more foods high in omega-3 fatty acids, antioxidants, and vitamin D. Nutrition may not be able to stop the aging process entirely, but it may make a huge difference in the quality of life for seniors by reducing inflammation and improving their joint health.

Foods that may exacerbate inflammation and joint pain.

Through my investigation, I have come to a better grasp of the ways in which my parents' dietary choices may have affected their joint health and the resulting pain and inflammation.

It's clear that my parents' love of sweets contributed to their ongoing battles with joint discomfort. My mother's joint pain may have been caused, in part, by her penchant for sweets and sugary drinks. Inflammation, like that caused by refined carbohydrates, can make joint discomfort seem much worse. Let's pretend that my mum is eating a sugary pastry, one of her all-time favorite desserts. She enjoyed the flavor, but it's possible her body was reacting negatively to the sugar in it. This could have started a vicious cycle of inflammation and joint pain that limited her ability to go about her normal life.

My dad may have experienced the negative effects of trans fats due to his penchant for fast food and packaged snacks. Fried foods and processed snacks are notorious for containing trans fats, which are known to cause inflammation. It's possible that his frequent eating of such meals triggered the aches in his joints. Think picture my dad opening a bag of chips. He was unwittingly putting trans fats into his body. The accumulation of pain and discomfort could have been caused by an inflammatory response in his joints, which the consumption of these lipids could have prompted. It's possible that his penchant for these meals contributed to the difficulties he experienced as a result of joint inflammation.

My mom and dad both suffered from joint pain in their latter years, and I believe that eating too many processed foods was a contributing factor. Inflammation may be exacerbated by the harmful fats and chemicals that are commonly found in these foods. Think about the pre-packaged snacks and microwave dinners that people resorted to on hectic days.

Imagine my mom and dad eating a microwave dinner. Their joint health may have suffered as a result of these options' convenience. It's possible that the preservatives and bad fats in these foods triggered ongoing inflammation in their joints, causing pain and restricting their range of motion.

My parents' experiences have taught me that certain food choices might exacerbate joint discomfort and inflammation. Perhaps unwittingly, the refined carbohydrates, trans fats, and processed meals they ate added to their discomfort. My parents could have made better decisions for their overall health if they had known about these links. This is to warn you about a few potential pitfalls. I promised you some homeopathic treatments, and here they are! This is important, in my opinion, since I think your way of life has a bearing on

The importance of maintaining a healthy weight to reduce stress on joints

The complex mechanisms of our joints allow us to make literally thousands of movements every single day. However, these essential tissues can feel the strain of excess weight, which can cause pain and limitations in movement. Those dealing with joint troubles would do well to learn about the correlation between a healthy weight and less joint stress.

Seeing as how my parents were having trouble with joint pain, I made it my duty to help them maintain a healthy weight and lessen the strain on their bones and joints. This post describes the all-encompassing strategy I employed to aid my parents on their path to better joint health.

The first step on this path was teaching my parents about the complex connection between being overweight and experiencing joint discomfort. I explained, both in person and in written form, how excess weight increases the severity of joint pain and hampers mobility. This realization served as the cornerstone of their weight-management determination. I suggested that my parents practice mindful eating to foster long-lasting improvement in their relationship with food.

I helped them tune into their internal cues for hunger and fullness so they could make more informed decisions about what and how much to eat. To achieve their weight loss targets, they were also careful of the quality of the food they ate.

We worked together to create a nutritious and well-rounded eating plan. I harped on the value of eating a diet rich in protein, fiber, complex carbohydrates, fruits, vegetables, and healthy fats. They were able to lose weight while still getting enough calories to fuel their bodies because of this strategy. They attribute most of their success with weight loss to their increased water intake. I hammered home how critical it is to keep drinking water regularly throughout the day. This helped their metabolism and kept them from eating too much, both of which are necessary for successful weight management.

The inclusion of specialized physical activity within their plan was crucial. We discussed activities like fast walking, swimming, and light yoga that are easier on the body. Not only did they help them burn calories, but they also kept their joints limber without putting too much stress on them. Motivating oneself to lose weight effectively required setting reasonable objectives. By setting attainable goals, they were able to feel a growing sense of pride as they crossed each one off their list.

Positive reinforcement and motivation were provided by commemorating even the smallest of achievements.

I joined them on their adventure after realizing the value of having a strong group of people behind you. My constant support, empathy, and insistence on personal responsibility were always appreciated. Our combined efforts helped them see their weight loss as a team effort, which strengthened their resolve. We were able to track their progress and make 'any required adjustments to their weight-management strategy thanks to the regular check-ins. This flexible method kept techniques from becoming ineffective by adjusting to new circumstances.

I helped my parents use relaxation strategies and mindfulness practices to address the emotional side effects of their weight loss efforts. These resources helped them develop effective stress management skills, curb emotional eating, and set themselves up for long-term success.

My efforts to help my parents achieve weight loss success were comprehensive. They not only lost weight but also felt better in their joints after engaging in a program of education, mindful eating, balanced diet, individualized physical exercise, and constant encouragement.

The change was not limited to the body; it also boosted mood and paved the way for longer-term improvements in things like bone and cartilage health.

Exercise and Physical Activity

Low-impact exercises and Instructions to follow

Low-impact exercises are gentle on the joints and provide a safe and effective way for seniors to maintain their fitness and overall health without putting excessive stress on their bodies. These exercises can help improve cardiovascular health, flexibility, strength, balance, and coordination, all of which are important for maintaining an active and independent lifestyle as we age. Low-impact exercises are particularly suitable for seniors, as they minimize the risk of injury and discomfort.

Walking

Benefits: Cardiovascular health, leg strength, balance.

➤ Find a safe and level area to walk.

➤ Stand up straight with shoulders relaxed and arms swinging naturally.

➤ Take a step forward with your right foot, heel-to-toe, and roll through the foot.

> Repeat with the left foot.

> Start with 10-15 minutes and gradually increase duration as comfortable.

Swimming

Benefits: Full-body workout, joint flexibility, cardiovascular fitness.

> Choose a pool with a comfortable temperature.

> Use a flotation device if needed.

> Practice gentle strokes, such as the breaststroke or sidestroke, to reduce impact on joints.

> Focus on smooth and controlled movements.

> Start with short sessions and gradually increase time in the water.

Cycling (Stationary or Recumbent)

Benefits: Leg strength, cardiovascular health, joint mobility.

> Adjust the bike seat and handlebars for proper alignment.

> Start pedaling at a comfortable pace.

- ➤ Maintain an even and controlled pedal stroke.

- ➤ Pay attention to your posture, keeping your back straight.

- ➤ Start with 10-15 minutes and work your way up.

Tai Chi

Benefits: Balance, flexibility, stress reduction.

- ➤ Find a quiet and open space.

- ➤ Follow a Tai Chi routine that focuses on slow, flowing movements.

- ➤ Concentrate on your breathing and staying relaxed.

- ➤ Start with a beginner's routine and gradually progress to more advanced forms.

Yoga

Benefits: Flexibility, balance, stress relief.

- ➤ Choose a beginner-friendly yoga routine.

- ➤ Use a yoga mat for cushioning and traction.

- ➤ Follow the instructor's guidance for each pose, moving slowly and mindfully.

> Focus on breathing deeply and maintaining proper alignment.

Seated Leg Lifts

Benefits: Leg strength, flexibility.

> Sit on a sturdy chair with feet flat on the floor.

> Lift your right leg straight out, extending it in front of you.

> Hold for a few seconds, then lower the leg.

> Repeat with the left leg.

> Aim for 10-15 repetitions on each leg.

Arm Raises

Benefits: Shoulder mobility, upper body strength.

> Sit or stand with proper posture.

> Hold a light weight in each hand or use your own body weight.

> Raise your arms out to the sides at shoulder height.

> Lower your arms back down slowly.

> Perform 10-15 repetitions.

Standing Heel Raises

Benefits: Calf strength, balance.

> ➢ Stand behind a sturdy chair, holding onto it for support.

> ➢ Slowly raise your heels off the ground, lifting onto your tiptoes.

> ➢ Hold for a moment, then lower your heels back down.

> ➢ Aim for 10-15 repetitions.

Leg Extensions

Benefits: Leg strength, balance.

> ➢ Sit on a chair with your back straight and feet flat on the floor.

> ➢ Lift one leg straight out in front of you, keeping the knee straight.

> ➢ Hold for a moment, then lower the leg.

> ➢ Repeat with the other leg.

> ➢ Perform 10-15 repetitions on each leg.

Wall Push-Ups

Benefits: Upper body strength.

> ➢ Stand facing a wall, about arm's length away.

> ➢ Place your hands on the wall at shoulder height and slightly wider than shoulder-width apart.

> ➢ Lean forward and bend your elbows, lowering your chest toward the wall.

> ➢ Push back to the starting position.

> ➢ Perform 10-15 repetitions.

Chair Yoga

Benefits: Flexibility, balance, relaxation.

> ➢ Sit in a sturdy chair with your back straight and feet flat on the floor.

> ➢ Follow a chair yoga routine, which includes gentle stretches and poses.

> ➢ Pay attention to your breath and hold each pose for a few breaths.

> ➢ This practice can help improve mobility and reduce stiffness.

Water Aerobics

Benefits: Cardiovascular fitness, joint support, muscle toning.

> ➤ Join a water aerobics class in a pool.

> ➤ Follow the instructor's lead for low-impact exercises in the water.

> ➤ The buoyancy of the water reduces stress on joints while providing resistance.

Resistance Band Exercises

Benefits: Muscle strength, joint stability.

> ➤ Secure a resistance band under your feet and hold the ends in your hands.

> ➤ Perform bicep curls by bending your elbows and lifting the bands towards your shoulders.

> ➤ Engage in leg lifts by placing the band around your ankles and lifting one leg at a time.

> ➤ These exercises can be tailored to different fitness levels.

Stationary Rowing

Benefits: Cardiovascular health, upper and lower body strength.

> ➤ Use a stationary rowing machine if available.

> ➤ Sit down, hold the handles, and start pulling back using your arms and legs.

> ➤ Push forward to return to the starting position.

> ➤ This exercise provides a full-body workout without high impact.

Stationary Marching

Benefits: Cardiovascular fitness, leg strength.

> ➤ Stand in a comfortable place.

> ➤ March in place by lifting one knee at a time, swinging your arms naturally.

> ➤ This simple exercise can help improve heart health and leg muscle tone.

Leg Circles

Benefits: Hip mobility, core engagement.

> - Lie on your back on a mat with your legs extended.

> - Lift one leg a few inches off the ground and start making small circles with your toes.

> - Perform clockwise circles for a set number of repetitions, then switch to counterclockwise circles.

> - This exercise helps with hip flexibility and stability.

Ankle Alphabet

Benefits: Ankle mobility, joint health.

> - Sit comfortably in a chair with your feet off the ground.

> - Pretend your toes are a pen and "write" the alphabet in the air with your ankle.

> - Repeat with the other foot.

> - This exercise promotes ankle flexibility and can help prevent stiffness.

Standing Knee Extensions

Benefits: Leg strength, balance.

> ➢ Stand upright, holding onto a sturdy surface if needed.

> ➢ Lift one knee towards your chest, extending the leg fully.

> ➢ Lower the leg back down with control.

> ➢ Alternate legs and perform 10-15 repetitions on each side.

Neck Stretches

Benefits: Neck flexibility, tension relief.

> ➢ Sit or stand with a straight posture.

> ➢ Slowly tilt your head to one side, bringing your ear towards your shoulder.

> ➢ Hold for a gentle stretch, then switch to the other side.

> ➢ You can also gently rotate your head left and right to stretch different neck muscles.

Finger and Hand Exercises

Benefits: Hand dexterity, joint health.

> ➤ Sit comfortably with your hands resting on a table.

> ➤ Open and close your hands, spreading your fingers as wide as possible and then making a fist.

> ➤ Rotate your wrists and perform simple finger taps on the table.

> ➤ These exercises can help maintain hand strength and coordination.

The benefits of strength training to support joint function

Strength training is a valuable component of fitness, especially for seniors, as it offers numerous benefits for joint health and overall well-being. As your parents age, their joint function can naturally decline, leading to issues like stiffness, reduced mobility, and increased risk of injury. Engaging in a well-designed strength training program can counteract these effects and provide the following benefits:

Improved Muscle Strength

Strength training helps to build and maintain muscle mass, which plays a crucial role in supporting joints. Strong muscles around joints provide better stability, reducing the risk of falls and joint-related injuries.

Enhanced Joint Stability

Strengthening the muscles around joints, such as the knees and hips, increases their stability. This can alleviate pressure on the joint itself and help maintain proper alignment during movement.

Increased Bone Density

Weight-bearing strength exercises promote bone health by stimulating bone density improvement. This is particularly important for seniors, as it can reduce the risk of osteoporosis and fractures.

Enhanced Range of Motion

Strength training through a full range of motion helps maintain and improve joint flexibility. Well-functioning joints with good mobility are less prone to stiffness and discomfort.

Cartilage Support

While strength training doesn't directly impact cartilage, it helps enhance overall joint function, which can indirectly support the health of the cartilage by maintaining proper joint mechanics.

Pain Management

Strengthening the muscles around joints can help distribute stress more evenly, potentially reducing pain associated with joint conditions like arthritis.

Strength Training Exercises and Instruction to follow

When recommending strength training exercises for seniors, it's essential to focus on low-impact, joint-friendly movements. Here are some exercises that your parents or you can consider incorporating into your or their routine:

Leg Pres

Benefits: Builds leg strength to support hip and knee joints.

How To

> Use a leg press machine or resistance bands.

- ➢ Sit down with your feet flat and shoulder-width apart.

- ➢ Push the weight or bands away using your legs, then return to the starting position.

Seated Rows

Benefits: Strengthens upper back muscles, supporting good posture and shoulder joint stability.

How To

- ➢ Sit down at a rowing machine or use resistance bands.

- ➢ Hold the handles and pull them toward your torso, squeezing your shoulder blades together.

- ➢ Slowly release the handles back to the starting position.

Wall Squats

Benefits: Builds lower body strength, especially in the quadriceps and glutes.

How To

- ➢ Stand with your back against a wall and your feet about hip-width apart.

➢ Slide down the wall into a squatting position, keeping your knees over your ankles.

➢ Hold for a few seconds, then push through your heels to return to standing.

Bicep Curls

Benefits: Increases arm strength, supporting elbow and shoulder joints.

How To

➢ Hold a light dumbbell in each hand, arms by your sides.

➢ Curl the dumbbells toward your shoulders, keeping your elbows close to your body.

➢ Lower the dumbbells back down with control.

Leg Extensions

Benefits: Strengthens quadriceps muscles to support knee joint function.

How To

➢ Sit on a leg extension machine or use resistance bands.

➢ Lift one leg straight out in front of you, extending your knee.

> Lower the leg back down, then switch to the other leg.

Chest Press

Benefits: Builds chest and shoulder muscles, promoting better upper body joint stability.

How To

> Use a chest press machine or resistance bands.

> Push the handles away from your chest, then bring them back toward you.

> Focus on controlled movements and proper form.

Bridge Exercise

Benefits: Strengthens glutes and core muscles, supporting hip and lower back joints.

How To

> Lie on your back with knees bent and feet flat on the floor.

> Lift your hips toward the ceiling, creating a straight line from shoulders to knees.

> Lower your hips back down with control.

Shoulder Press

Benefits: Increases shoulder strength, improving joint stability.

How To

> Use dumbbells or resistance bands.

> Hold the weights at shoulder height, palms facing forward.

> Press the weights upward until your arms are fully extended, then lower them back down.

Plank

Benefits: Strengthens core muscles, supporting spine and hip joints.

How To

> Start in a push-up position, but with your weight supported on your forearms.

> Keep your body in a straight line from head to heels, engaging your core.

> Hold this position for as long as comfortable, focusing on proper alignment.

Standing Calf Raises

Benefits: Builds calf muscles, supporting ankle and lower leg joints.

<u>How To</u>

> ➤ Stand with your feet flat on the ground.

> ➤ Rise up onto the balls of your feet, then lower your heels back down.

> ➤ Hold onto a sturdy surface for balance if needed.

Before starting any strength training program, it's crucial for your parents to consult a healthcare professional to ensure that the exercises are safe and appropriate for their individual health conditions. A fitness professional can also provide guidance on proper technique and help tailor the exercises to their specific needs and goals. Gradually increasing the weight and intensity of the exercises over time will allow them to experience the benefits of improved joint function and overall strength.

Flexibility exercises and their impact on joint mobility

Flexibility exercises are designed to improve the range of motion of your joints and muscles. Regular flexibility training can help enhance joint mobility, reduce muscle stiffness, and improve overall functional movement. It's important to note that flexibility exercises should be performed safely and gradually, as overstretching or improper technique can lead to injuries.

Benefits of flexibility exercises include:

> Increased joint range of motion.

> Improved posture and balance.

> Reduced muscle tension and discomfort.

> Enhanced athletic performance.

> Prevention of injuries related to muscle imbalances.

Flexibility Exercises and Instruction to follow

Here are 10 flexibility exercises that you or your parents can incorporate into a regular stretching routine. Remember to perform these exercises gently and gradually, and avoid pushing yourself too hard.

Neck Stretch

Gently tilt your head to the side, bringing your ear towards your shoulder. Hold for 15-30 seconds on each side.

Shoulder Stretch

Extend one arm across your body and gently press it with your opposite hand. Hold for 15-30 seconds on each side.

Triceps Stretch

Raise one arm overhead and bend your elbow, bringing your hand down your back. Gently press the elbow with your opposite hand. Hold for 15-30 seconds on each side.

Chest Opener

Clasp your hands behind your back and gently lift your arms, opening up your chest. Hold for 15-30 seconds.

Quadriceps Stretch

Stand on one leg, bend the opposite knee, and grab your ankle. Gently pull your ankle towards your glutes. Hold for 15-30 seconds on each side.

Hamstring Stretch

Sit on the floor with one leg extended and the other leg bent, sole of the foot against the inner thigh. Reach toward your extended foot, keeping your back straight. Hold for 15-30 seconds on each side.

Groin Stretch

Sit on the floor, bring the soles of your feet together, and gently press your knees down towards the floor. Hold for 15-30 seconds.

Hip Flexor Stretch

Take a lunge position with one foot forward and the other foot back. Gently press your hips forward while keeping your back straight. Hold for 15-30 seconds on each side.

Standing Forward Fold

Stand with your feet hip-width apart and fold forward at the hips, letting your upper body hang. Bend your knees slightly if needed. Hold for 15-30 seconds.

Calf Stretch

Stand facing a wall, place your hands on the wall, and step one foot back while keeping it straight. Gently press the heel of the back foot toward the ground. Hold for 15-30 seconds on each side.

Remember to breathe deeply and relax into each stretch. If you or your parents have any pre-existing medical conditions or injuries, it's a good idea to consult a healthcare professional before starting a new flexibility routine.

CHAPTER THREE

Herbal Remedies and Supplements

My desire to aid my parents has also taken me into the field of herbal remedies, where I have uncovered a veritable treasure trove of natural solutions that have vastly enhanced their quality of life.

Turmeric was one of the first herbs I used when I needed a natural remedy. This colorful spice, which is high in the anti-inflammatory compound curcumin, really stood out. My mother and father's stiffness and movement both improved once they began included turmeric in their daily routine, either as a tasty supplement to meals or in relaxing cups of turmeric tea. Drinking hot tea became a soothing routine that helped ease my aching joints.

Our collection of herbal treatments quickly expanded to include ginger. We started using the pungent root for its medicinal benefits, including its ability to reduce inflammation and alleviate pain. Making a cup of ginger tea became a soothing ritual, and the rising steam appeared to carry away the persistent pain. My mom and dad's joint discomfort seemed to lessen with each sip, and they resumed doing things they had practically given up on because of it.

However, comfort came from more than just old favorites. As I dug deeper, I came across herbal supplements and alternative medicines like cat's claw and devil's claw. These mysterious plants, with their equally mysterious names, were able to effectively reduce inflammation. I found that my parents' joint pain lessened when they began including them in their daily routine. These herbs provided a mild but efficient method of pain management, whether in the form of properly measured pills or a soothing tea.

It was impossible to ignore the calming effects of topical treatments. Joint pain management became more targeted with the introduction of capsaicin creams loaded with the heat of chili peppers. The anti-inflammatory properties of eucalyptus oil, combined with a soothing massage, helped relieve the stress that had become a frequent companion. As I administered the calming ointments, I watched my parent's look soften, and I knew that I had done more than just relieve their agony.

The voyage was made easier and more hopeful with each natural treatment. Each plant contributed something to the puzzle of relieving my parents' joint discomfort, from the time-tested benefits of turmeric to the novelty of cat's claw. Herbal supplements are not a silver bullet, but they have helped my mom and dad tremendously.

One cup of tea and one calming treatment at a time, they provided a means of connection, exploration, and healing that has made a profound impact on their lives.

Common Herbal Remedies I Tried

Turmeric

<u>Ingredients</u>

> Turmeric root (containing curcumin)

<u>Preparation</u>

> Add 1 teaspoon of turmeric powder to boiling water, let it simmer for 10 minutes, strain, and optionally add honey or lemon.

<u>Targeted Joint Areas</u>

> Beneficial for inflammation and pain in various joints.

<u>Nutritional Composition</u>

> Rich in curcumin, an anti-inflammatory and antioxidant compound.

Ginger

Ingredients

> ➤ Fresh ginger root

Preparation

> ➤ Slice ginger and boil in water for 10-15 minutes, strain, and add honey or lemon.

Targeted Joint Areas

> ➤ Effective for reducing inflammation and pain across multiple joints.

Nutritional Composition

> ➤ Contains gingerol, with anti-inflammatory and pain-relieving properties.

Boswellia

Ingredients

> ➤ Resin from the Boswellia tree

Preparation

> ➤ Take Boswellia supplements by following recommended dosage on the product label.

Targeted Joint Areas

> Primarily used for inflammation and pain in the knees and hips.

Nutritional Composition

> Contains boswellic acids, which possess anti-inflammatory attributes.

Willow Bark

Ingredients

> Willow bark extract (salicin)

Preparation

> Consume willow bark which is available as tea, capsules, or tinctures; follow product label instructions.

Targeted Joint Areas

> Offers pain relief to various joints, including the back and knees.

Nutritional Composition

> Contains salicin, metabolized into salicylic acid akin to aspirin.

Devil's Claw

Ingredients

> ➤ Devil's claw root extract

Preparation

> ➤ Use Devil's Claw supplements and adhere to recommended dosage on the product label.

Targeted Joint Areas

> ➤ Alleviates inflammation and pain in the knees and lower back.

Nutritional Composition

> ➤ Contains harpagoside, a compound with potential anti-inflammatory effects.

Capsaicin

Ingredients

> ➤ Capsaicin extracted from chili peppers

Preparation

> ➤ Apply capsaicin creams: Topical application on affected joints; follow product label instructions.

<u>Targeted Joint Areas</u>

> Provides relief to joints such as fingers, wrists, and elbows.

<u>Nutritional Composition</u>

> Blocks pain signals and promotes local blood circulation.

Eucalyptus

<u>Ingredients</u>

> Eucalyptus essential oil

<u>Preparation</u>

> Dilute eucalyptus oil: Mix with a carrier oil for massages or add a few drops to a warm bath.

<u>Targeted Joint Areas</u>

> Beneficial for joint pain in various body areas.

<u>Nutritional Composition</u>

> Contains eucalyptol, with anti-inflammatory and analgesic effects.

Arnica

Ingredients

> Arnica flower extract

Preparation

> Apply Arnica gel/cream: Topical application on affected joints; follow product label instructions.

Targeted Joint Areas

> Commonly used for joint pain in knees, wrists, and ankles.

Nutritional Composition

> Contains helenalin, a compound with potential anti-inflammatory properties.

Stinging Nettle

Ingredients

> Stinging nettle leaves

Preparation

> Brew stinging nettle tea: Steep dried leaves in hot water for 10-15 minutes, then strain.

Targeted Joint Areas

> ➤ Addresses inflammation in various joints.

Nutritional Composition

> ➤ Rich in vitamins, minerals, and antioxidants.

White Willow Bark

Ingredients

> ➤ White willow bark extract (salicin)

Preparation

> ➤ Consume white willow bark: Available as tea, capsules, or tinctures; follow product label instructions.

Targeted Joint Areas

> ➤ Offers relief for joints such as hips and back.

Nutritional Composition

> ➤ Contains salicin, which offers pain-relieving effects.

Licorice Root

Ingredients

> ➤ Licorice root

Preparation

> ➤ Brew licorice root tea: Boil a teaspoon of dried licorice root in water for 10 minutes, strain, and enjoy.

Targeted Joint Areas

> ➤ Can help with inflammation in various joints.

Nutritional Composition

> ➤ Contains glycyrrhizin, which has anti-inflammatory properties.

Chamomile

Ingredients

> ➤ Chamomile flowers

Preparation

> ➤ Brew chamomile tea: Steep chamomile flowers in hot water for about 5 minutes, then strain and add honey if desired.

Targeted Joint Areas

 ➤ Mild anti-inflammatory effects can benefit various joints.

Nutritional Composition

 ➤ Contains antioxidants and anti-inflammatory compounds.

Olive Oil

Ingredients

 ➤ Extra virgin olive oil

Preparation

 ➤ Apply olive oil topically: Warm the oil slightly and massage it onto the affected joint.

Targeted Joint Areas

Can provide relief to joints like fingers, wrists, and elbows.

Nutritional Composition

Rich in monounsaturated fats and antioxidants.

Pine Bark Extract

<u>Ingredients</u>

> ➢ Extract from the bark of pine trees

<u>Preparation</u>

> ➢ Take pine bark supplements: Follow recommended dosage on the product label.

<u>Targeted Joint Areas</u>

> ➢ Used to alleviate joint pain and improve joint function.

<u>Nutritional Composition</u>

> ➢ Contains proanthocyanidins, potent antioxidants with potential anti-inflammatory effects.

Essential Oils and Aromatherapy

Essential oils that have shown potential for reducing joint pain and inflammation. Many essential oils have anti-inflammatory and pain-relieving properties. However, I will reiterate that you should see a doctor if you have been hurt, if you have a medical condition that can produce these symptoms, or if you have no idea what is causing the pain and inflammation. Let's jump right into the topic of using essential oils to treat aching joints and swelling.

Lavender Essential Oil

Lavender essential oil is a common ingredient in homes and businesses that want to foster a soothing atmosphere. This is due to the calming effects of lavender essential oil. This powerful oil, however, has many more applications besides that. Lavender essential oil has been shown to be effective in reducing joint inflammation due to its anti-inflammatory properties. Massage the diluted lavender essential oil into the afflicted joints or the inflammatory areas by mixing it with a carrier oil (such as coconut oil or jojoba oil). A few drops in a warm bath might also help you unwind.

Eucalyptus Essential Oil

Joint and muscular discomfort can be alleviated with the help of eucalyptus essential oil because of its therapeutic characteristics. The anti-inflammatory and antispasmodic qualities of eucalyptus essential oil are aided by its cooling and soothing aroma. A carrier oil and a few drops of eucalyptus essential oil will do wonders for aching muscles and joints. A few drops added to a diffuser can also help with breathing and pain relief.

Rosemary Essential Oil

Rosemary essential oil is another great option for people who suffer from inflammation or joint pain because it contains potent antioxidants and has pain-relieving and anti-inflammatory qualities. Apply a mixture of rosemary essential oil and carrier oil to the afflicted regions. A warm compress with a few drops of the oil added can provide localized relief to the joints.

Extract of Ginger

Zingibain, an anti-inflammatory component found in ginger essential oil, helps reduce muscle and joint swelling, inflammation, discomfort, and stiffness. Essential ginger oil has anti-inflammatory and analgesic characteristics that make it useful for relieving pain and enhancing mobility. Massage aching muscles and joints with a mixture of ginger essential oil and a carrier oil. You can also make a compress by adding a few drops of ginger oil to a warm, damp cloth and applying it to the affected region for a soothing warming sensation.

Essential Oil of Chamomile

You can do a lot with chamomile flowers. You can make a tea from them and use it for beauty treatments or to reduce the effects of a fever.

Chamomile's anti-inflammatory properties are enhanced in its essential oil form. Because of its relaxing properties, chamomile essential oil is excellent for easing anxious thoughts and promoting sound sleep. Chamomile essential oil, mixed with a carrier oil, can be massaged into sore joints for relief. A few drops in a warm bath before night might help you unwind and ease any aches or pains.

Marjoram Essential Oil

Traditional medicine relied on marjoram essential oil to alleviate pain from sprains, inflammation, stiffness, and spasms. That's because marjoram is so effective in relieving pain, fighting germs, and relaxing muscles. Joint and muscular discomfort can be alleviated with either pure marjoram essential oil or a mixture containing marjoram, lavender, Red Mandarin, and Mandarin Petitgrain, such as Renewed Calm mixture.

This concoction is ideal for relieving mild discomfort because it calms the nerves, soothes the muscles, and allows for a more restful night's sleep. Massage the afflicted regions with a mixture of marjoram essential oil and a carrier oil. You can increase its relaxing effects by combining it with other oils. You can also find comfort and relaxation by diffusing marjoram oil in your home.

Peppermint Essential Oil

Joint discomfort, pains, and inflammation can be alleviated with the help of peppermint, a hybrid mint plant that has been utilized for thousands of years. Because of the menthol content, this ancient herb has been used medicinally for thousands of years to alleviate symptoms of arthritis and other inflammatory conditions.

To alleviate heat, stress, and pain, menthol can be used as a cooling agent. Applying peppermint oil topically can have a dramatic, immediate effect on joint pain and inflammation. Peppermint essential oil, when mixed with a carrier oil and massaged into sore joints, provides both cooling relief and temporary relief from inflammation. Peppermint oil is potent and should be used with caution, especially around the eyes and cheeks.

Thyme Essential Oil

Because of its antiseptic characteristics, thyme, like peppermint, has been used for thousands of years in traditional medicine as an antidote for venom and poison. The primary component of thyme, thymol, can reduce inflammation and swelling. Joint pain and inflammation, as well as dysmenorrhea-related pain and inflammation, can all be helped by using thyme essential oil.

Applying a blend of thyme essential oil and a carrier oil to sore joints will help reduce swelling and pain. A few drops in a warm bath might also help you relax.

Essential Frankincense Oil

Frankincense essential oil, which comes from the Boswellia tree, is widely used as a stress and pain reliever. Topical application of frankincense essential oil, in combination with a carrier oil, has been shown to have analgesic effects.

However, it can be diffused for a better night's rest. Apply a mixture of frankincense essential oil and a carrier oil to your aching joints and massage. A few drops in a diffuser might help you unwind and feel at peace with your surroundings.

Lemongrass Essential Oil

Joint pain and inflammation are two common signs of arthritis, and lemongrass essential oil is a popular Ayurvedic remedy for both. Because of its astringent qualities, lemongrass oil has the ability to reduce inflammation and increase mobility after being absorbed by the body. Massage the diluted essential oil of lemongrass into the affected joints. Lemongrass oil has a refreshing scent and may have health advantages if diffused.

Wintergreen Essential Oil

Wintergreen essential oil, which is extracted from the leaves of a North American tree, has a long history of use in North America for the treatment of rheumatism, back pain, joint discomfort, and headaches. Wintergreen essential oil is useful for relieving joint and muscle pain since it contains methyl salicylate, a molecule with similar attributes and properties to aspirin. Apply a solution of wintergreen essential oil diluted in a carrier oil to the affected regions. Due to its potency, it should be used with caution.

Never put on open wounds or consume.

Cayenne Pepper Essential Oil

Capsaicin, found in cayenne pepper, is a painkiller and inflammation fighter. Cayenne pepper essential oil contains similar characteristics, making it useful for treating inflammation and joint discomfort. Cayenne pepper essential oil, diluted in a carrier oil, can be massaged into aching joints for relief. Be wary, as cayenne oil has the potential to be quite fiery.

CHAPTER FOUR

Mind-Body Practices

Breathing Management for Pain

The root of most relaxation techniques is a simple action we make day in and day out: breathing. Your breath is a powerful tool you can use at home to help manage pain, soothe stress and calm restlessness.

Diaphragmatic Breathing

> ➢ Sit or lie down comfortably.

> ➢ Place one hand on your chest and the other on your abdomen.

> ➢ Inhale deeply through your nose, letting your abdomen rise.

> ➢ Exhale slowly through pursed lips, allowing your abdomen to fall.

> ➢ Helps improve oxygen flow and reduces tension, benefiting joint pain.

Inhaling deeply through the nose while allowing the abdomen to rise engages the diaphragm and enhances oxygen intake. This increased oxygen flow supports tissue healing and reduces joint discomfort.

4-7-8 Breathing

➢ Sit or lie down comfortably.

➢ Inhale through your nose for a count of 4.

➢ Hold your breath for a count of 7.

➢ Exhale through your mouth for a count of 8.

➢ Promotes relaxation and decreases stress, which can alleviate joint pain.

The extended exhalation in 4-7-8 breathing triggers the body's relaxation response, calming the nervous system. This reduction in stress directly eases tension around joints, promoting relief from pain.

Box Breathing

➢ Sit comfortably with your back straight.

➢ Inhale slowly through your nose for a count of 4.

➢ Hold your breath for a count of 4.

➢ Exhale slowly through your mouth for a count of 4.

➢ Pause for a count of 4 before repeating.

Enhances mindfulness and reduces muscle tension, benefiting joint discomfort. Box breathing fosters mindfulness and relaxation, diminishing muscle tightness often associated with joint pain. By alleviating muscle tension, this exercise indirectly provides relief to the affected joints.

Alternate Nostril Breathing

> Sit in a comfortable position.

> Use your thumb to close off your right nostril, inhale through the left.

> Close off the left nostril with your ring finger, exhale through the right.

> Inhale through the right nostril, then close it off and exhale through the left.

Helps balance energy and relaxes the nervous system, aiding joint pain management. Balancing the energy flow through alternate nostril breathing soothes the nervous system. As stress levels decrease, joint pain is mitigated due to the interconnection between stress and pain perception.

Pursed Lip Breathing

> Sit comfortably with your back straight.

> Inhale through your nose for a count of 2.

➢ Pucker your lips as if you're about to blow out candles.

➢ Exhale gently through pursed lips for a count of 4.

Reduces the work of breathing and promotes relaxation, relieving joint discomfort. Pursed lip breathing prolongs exhalation, ensuring better oxygen exchange. This technique aids in minimizing joint inflammation by improving circulation and oxygen supply to affected areas.

Deep Belly Breathing

➢ Lie down comfortably on your back.

➢ Place your hands on your abdomen.

➢ Inhale deeply through your nose, expanding your belly.

➢ Exhale slowly through your mouth, letting your belly fall.

Enhances oxygen exchange and encourages relaxation, aiding joint pain. The expanded inhalation and complete exhalation of deep belly breathing stimulate the relaxation response. By reducing stress-related tension, joint pain is managed more effectively.

Lion's Breath

- ➤ Sit comfortably with your back straight.

- ➤ Inhale deeply through your nose.

- ➤ Exhale forcefully through your mouth while sticking out your tongue and making a "ha" sound.

Reduces tension in the face and neck muscles, which can indirectly help with joint discomfort. Releasing tension from the face and neck through lion's breath indirectly benefits joint pain. Relaxed facial muscles can lead to an overall reduction in muscle tension and joint discomfort.

Equal Breathing

- ➤ Sit or lie down comfortably.

- ➤ Inhale through your nose for a count of 4.

- ➤ Exhale through your nose for a count of 4.

Promotes calmness and relaxation, potentially reducing joint pain. Equal breathing establishes equilibrium within the body, fostering a balanced environment for joint healing. The resulting relaxation response aids in mitigating joint pain.

Humming Bee Breath (Bhramari)

- ➢ Sit comfortably with your eyes closed.

- ➢ Place your thumbs on your ear cartilage and your fingers over your eyes.

- ➢ Inhale deeply through your nose.

- ➢ Exhale while making a humming sound like a bee.

This can have a soothing effect on the nervous system, indirectly helping with joint discomfort. The soothing effect of humming bee breath extends to the nervous system. By promoting relaxation, this exercise indirectly contributes to easing joint pain.

Resonant Breathing

- ➢ Sit or lie down comfortably.

- ➢ Inhale naturally and exhale naturally.

- ➢ As you breathe, count how many heartbeats it takes for each inhalation and exhalation.

- ➢ Aim for a 5:5 or 6:6 rhythm (inhale for a count of 5 or 6 heartbeats, exhale for the same).

Encourages heart rate variability and relaxation, which can assist in managing joint pain.

Resonant breathing's impact on heart rate variability directly influences stress reduction. A calmer state of being contributes to decreased muscle tension and reduced joint pain.

Three-Part Breath (Dirga Swasam Pranayama)

> ➢ Lie down comfortably on your back.

> ➢ Place one hand on your chest and the other on your abdomen.

> ➢ Inhale deeply, expanding your belly, then your ribcage, and finally your chest.

> ➢ Exhale in reverse order: chest, ribcage, belly.

> ➢ Promotes deep relaxation and mindful awareness, indirectly benefiting joint pain.

Relaxing Breath (4-2-6-2)

> ➢ Sit or lie down comfortably.

> ➢ Inhale through your nose for a count of 4.

> ➢ Hold your breath for a count of 2.

> ➢ Exhale through your mouth for a count of 6.

> ➢ Pause without inhaling for a count of 2.

Encourages relaxation and stress reduction, potentially alleviating joint discomfort.

CHAPTER FIVE

Heat and Cold Therapy

Heat and cold therapy are commonly used methods to manage joint pain. Applying heat can help relax muscles, improve blood circulation, and ease stiffness in joints. Cold therapy, on the other hand, can reduce inflammation and numb the area, providing temporary pain relief. Alternating between heat and cold can sometimes be effective for certain conditions, as it helps improve blood flow while reducing inflammation.

Heat Therapy helps relax muscles, improves flexibility, and increases blood flow, which can alleviate joint pain. While cold therapy reduces inflammation and numbs the area, providing pain relief, especially after injuries.

Proper Techniques for Using Hot and Cold Packs Safely

➤ Heat Packs: Use a warm, not hot, pack for around 15-20 minutes at a time. Make sure to place a cloth between the pack and your skin to avoid burns.

➤ Cold Packs: Apply a cold pack wrapped in a thin cloth for about 15-20 minutes at a time.

Avoid applying directly to the skin to prevent frostbite.

Acupuncture and Acupressure

Acupuncture and acupressure are traditional techniques rooted in Chinese medicine. Acupuncture involves inserting thin needles into specific points on the body, while acupressure involves applying pressure to these points. Both techniques are believed to stimulate energy pathways, known as meridians, to promote pain relief and healing.

Mechanisms of Acupuncture and Acupressure

Acupuncture: Needles stimulate nerves, triggering the release of endorphins (natural painkillers) and promoting better blood flow.

Acupressure: Pressure on acupoints can release muscle tension, improve circulation, and stimulate the body's natural healing processes.

Qualified Practitioners for Acupuncture and Acupressure

Seek practitioners who are licensed and trained in acupuncture or acupressure. They should have proper training, certification, and a solid understanding of anatomy and traditional Chinese medicine principles.

Hydrotherapy and Balneotherapy

Hydrotherapy involves using water for therapeutic purposes, while balneotherapy specifically utilizes mineral-rich water for healing. These techniques have been used for centuries to alleviate joint pain and promote relaxation.

Hot Springs and Mineral Baths

Hot springs and mineral baths contain minerals like sulfur, magnesium, and calcium that are believed to have healing properties. Immersing in these waters can soothe joint pain, reduce muscle tension, and promote overall well-being.

Precautions for Seniors in Hydrotherapy

Seniors should consult their healthcare provider before engaging in hydrotherapy, especially if they have underlying health conditions. The water temperature should be comfortable, not too hot, to avoid overheating. Adequate supervision and support are essential, and seniors should ease into hydrotherapy to prevent falls or accidents.

CONCLUSION

As we've journeyed through the corridors of this book, we've explored the intricate landscape of joint pain and the possibilities that lie within the embrace of nature. The pages before you stand as a testament to the resilience of the human spirit and the profound wisdom passed down through generations. The remedies shared within these chapters are not mere elixirs; they are the embodiment of time-tested truths that intertwine seamlessly with our quest for healing.

As the sun sets on these words, remember that the pursuit of relief from joint pain is not a solitary venture. It's a harmonious symphony of tradition and innovation, where the soothing touch of natural remedies dances alongside the advancements of modern medicine. Whether you choose the well-trodden path or forge a new one, know that you're never alone in this journey.

May the knowledge gleaned from these pages empower you to stride with renewed vigor, to reclaim those once-effortless activities, and to revel in the joy of mobility. Let this book be a companion on your path to wellness, a guiding light in times of discomfort, and a source of hope for the years yet to come.

Here's to a future where joint pain is not an insurmountable obstacle, but a chapter in the grand tale of a life lived fully and abundantly.